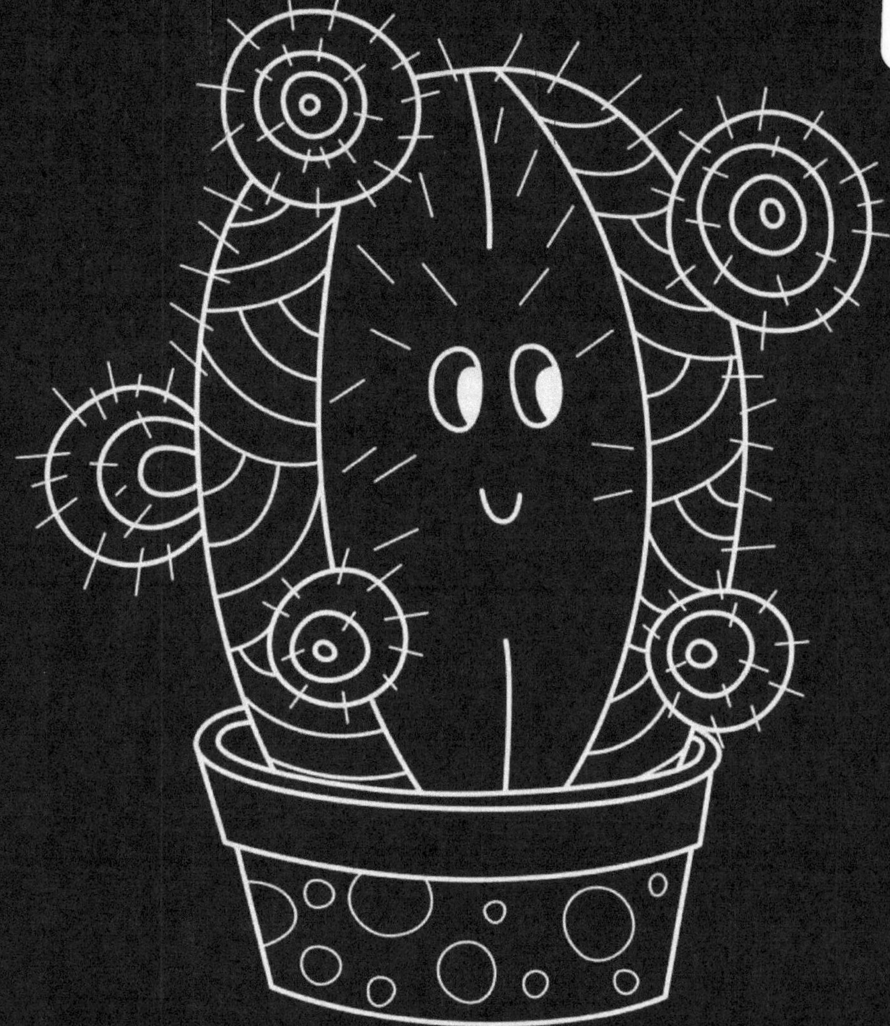

TINY CACTUS PUBLISHING

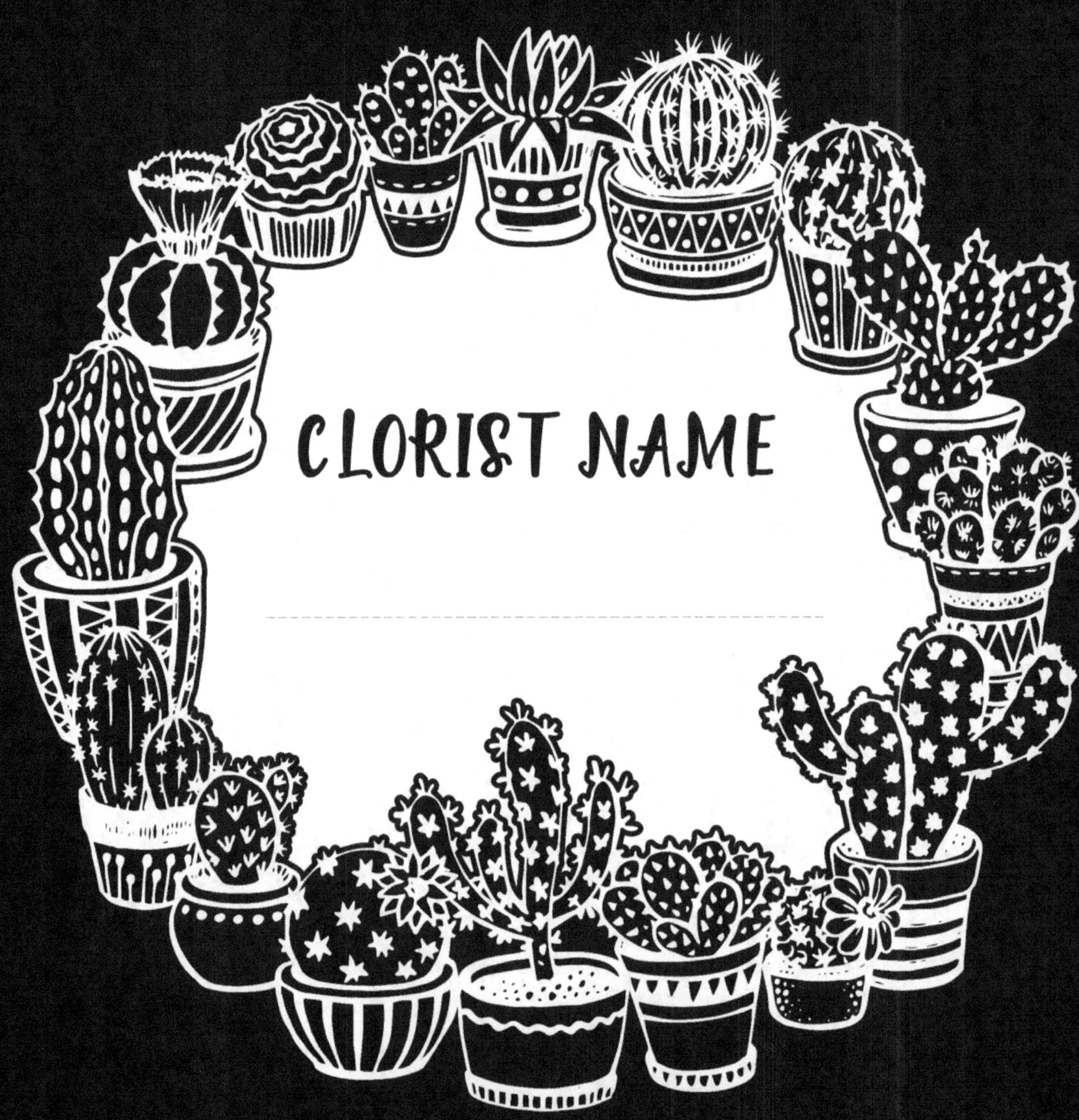
CLORIST NAME

TEST PAGE

PREPARE YOUR COLOR

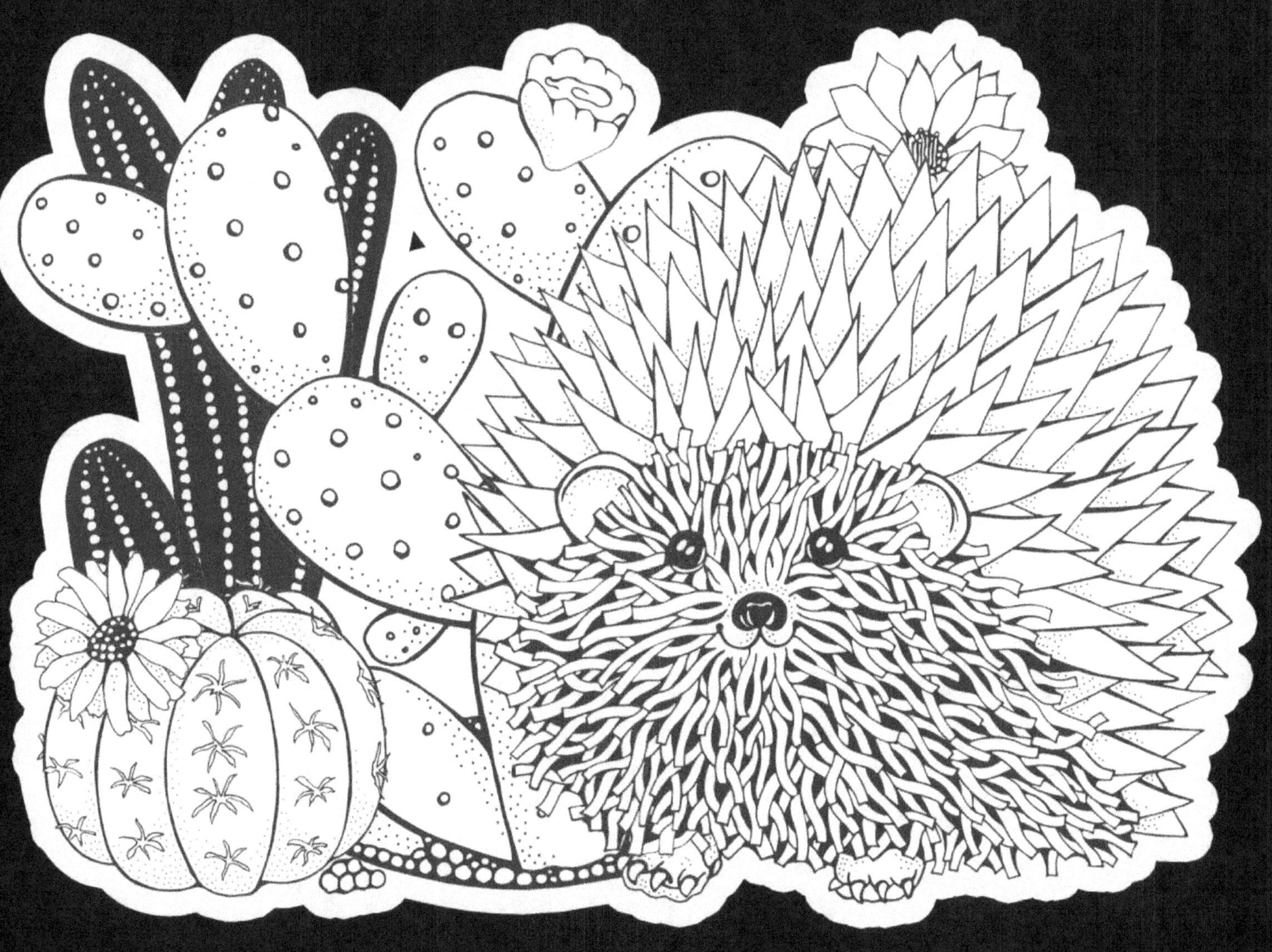

WARM UP !!

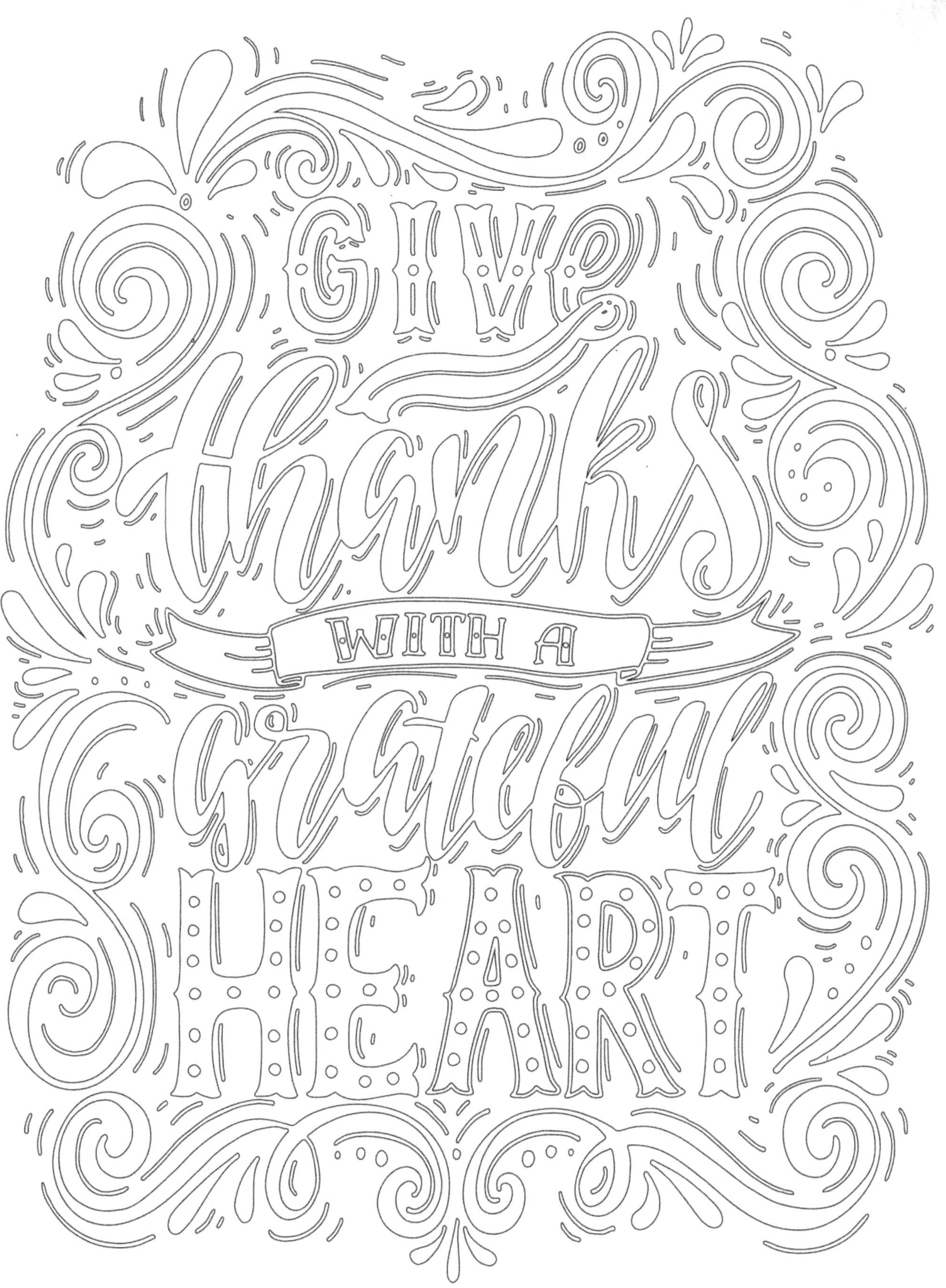

GIVE
thanks
WITH A
grateful
HEART

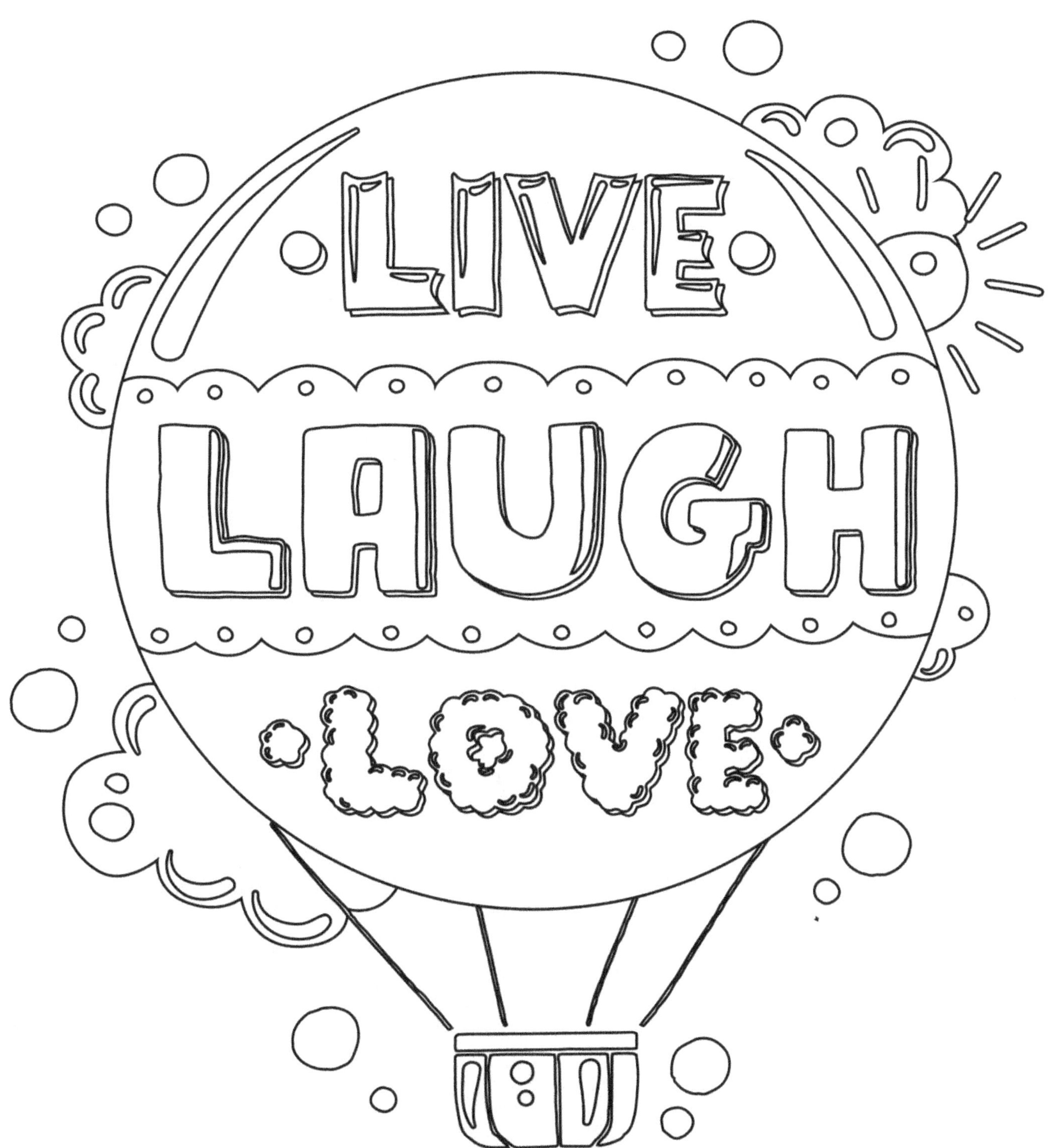

LIVE
LAUGH
·LOVE·

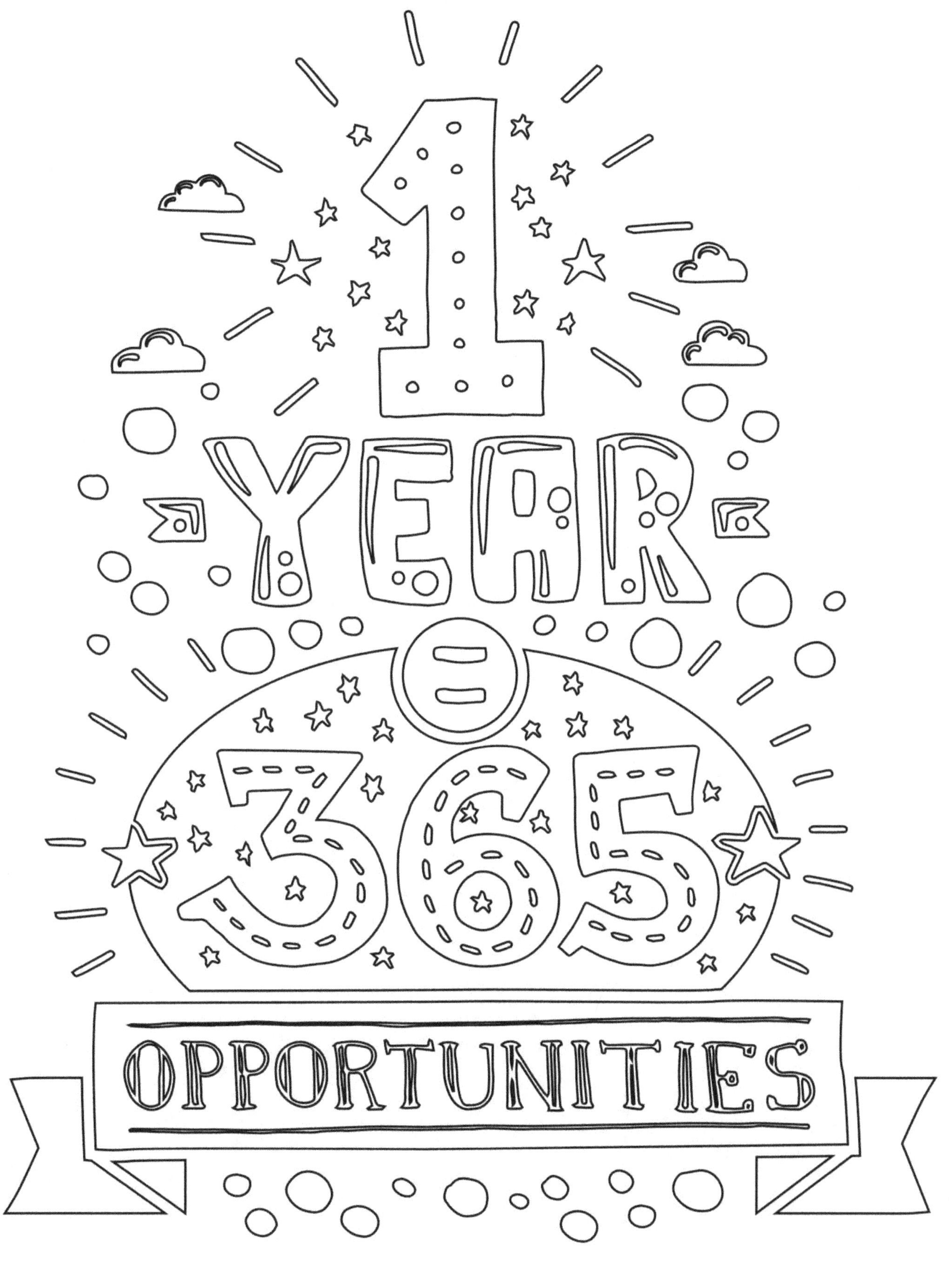
1
YEAR
=
365
OPPORTUNITIES

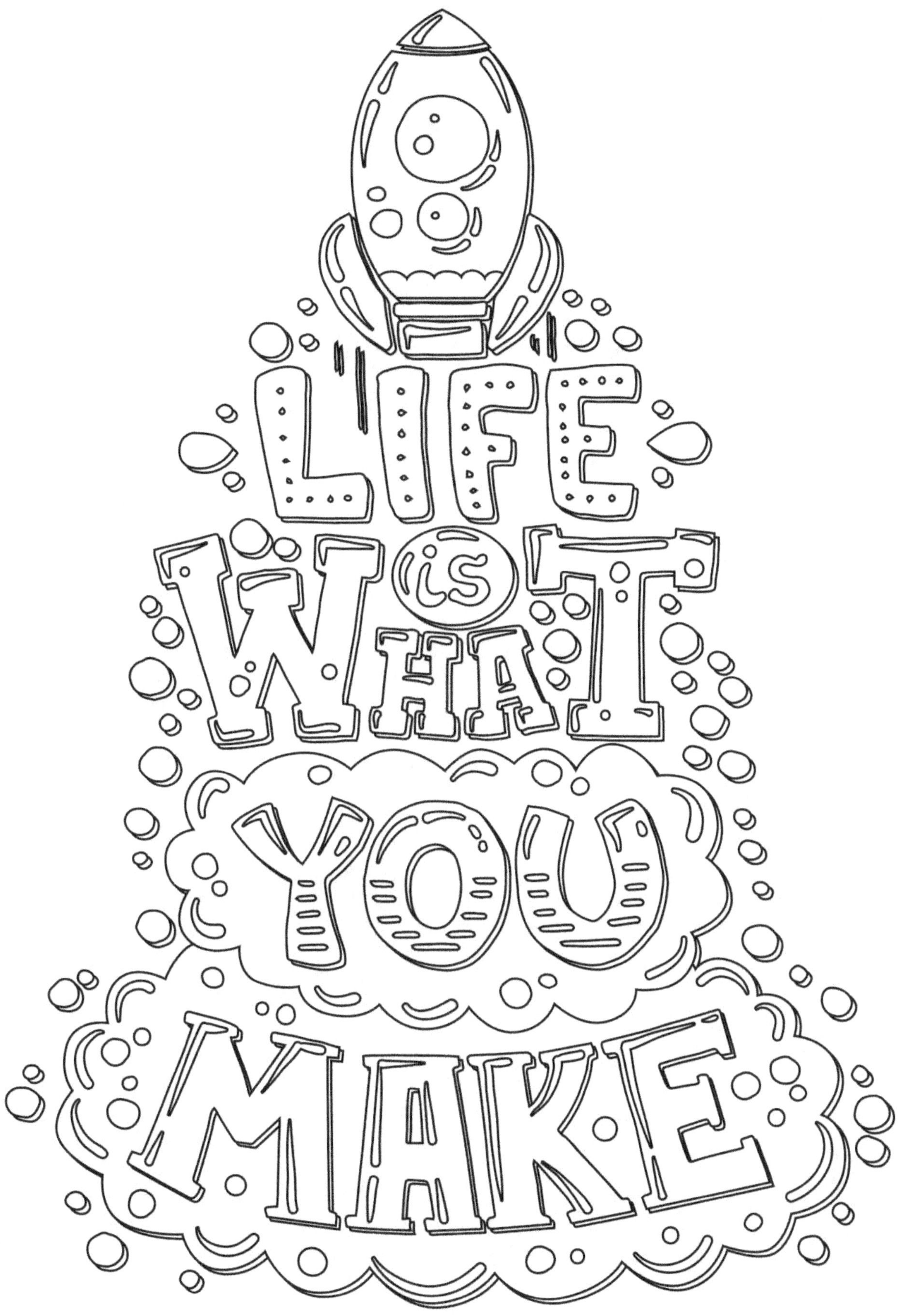

LIFE
IS
WHAT
YOU
MAKE

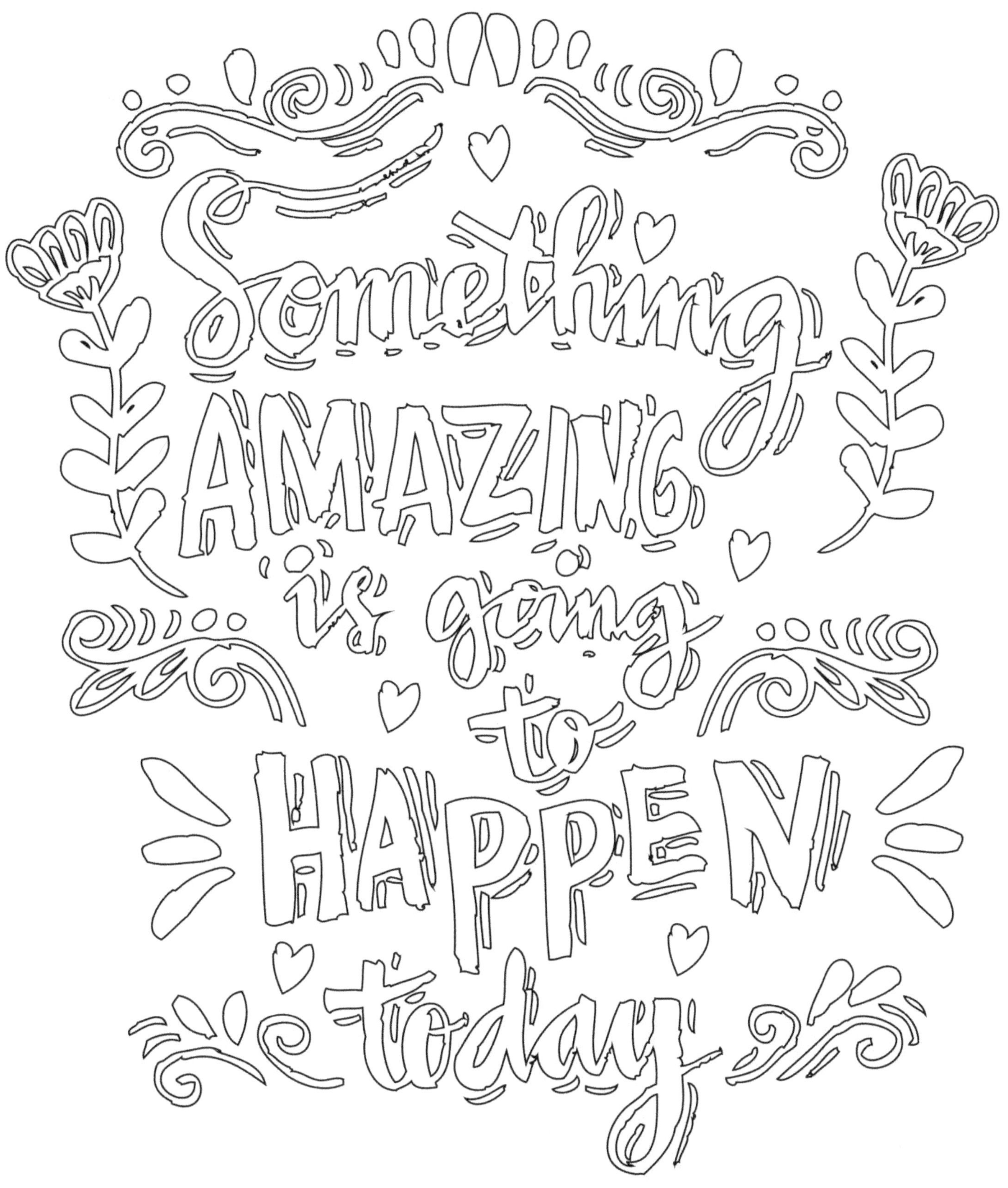

Something
AMAZING
is going
to
HAPPEN
today

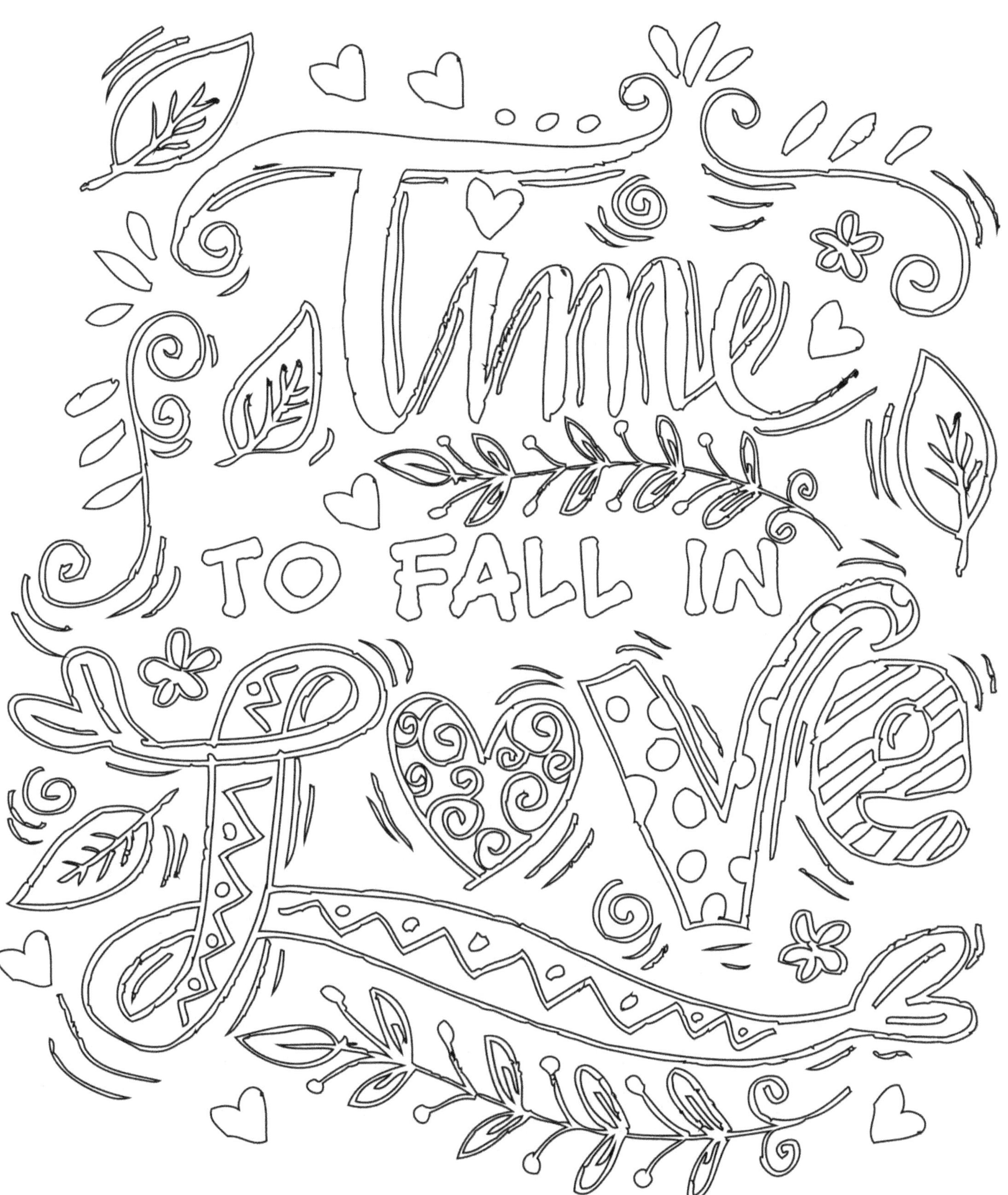

Time
TO FALL IN
Love

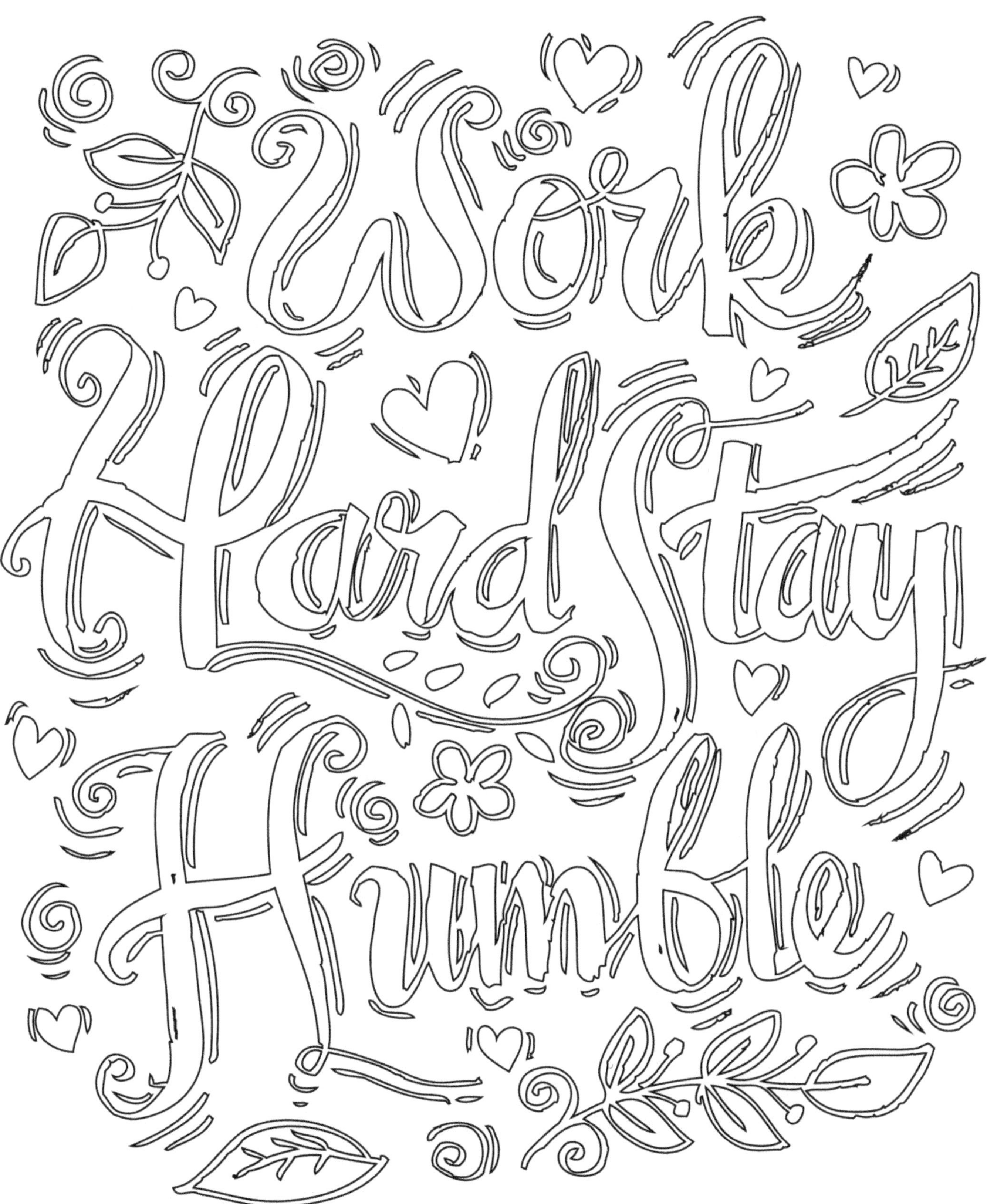
Work Hard Stay Humble

today is the PERFECT day of my life

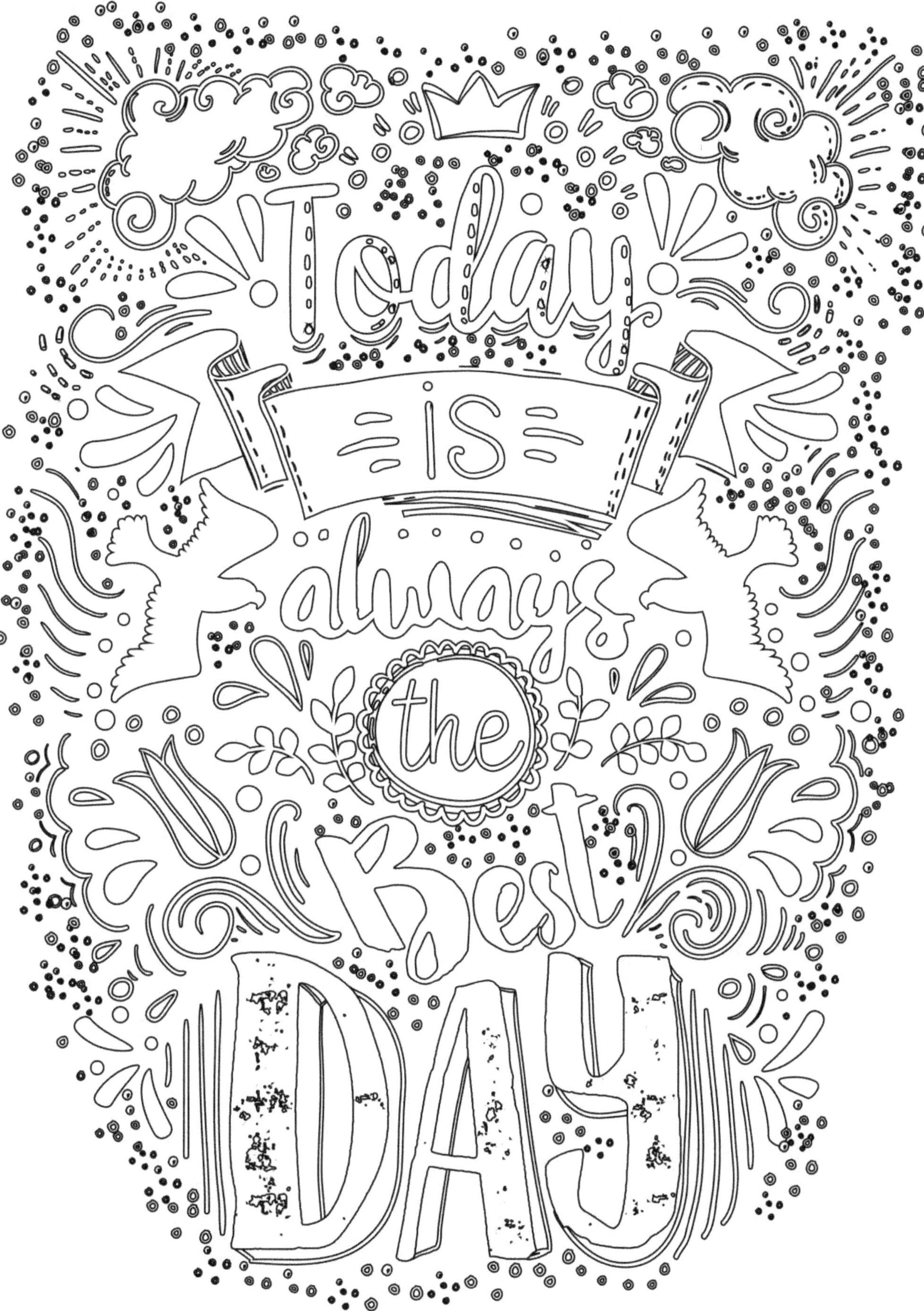

Today
IS
always
the
Best
DAY

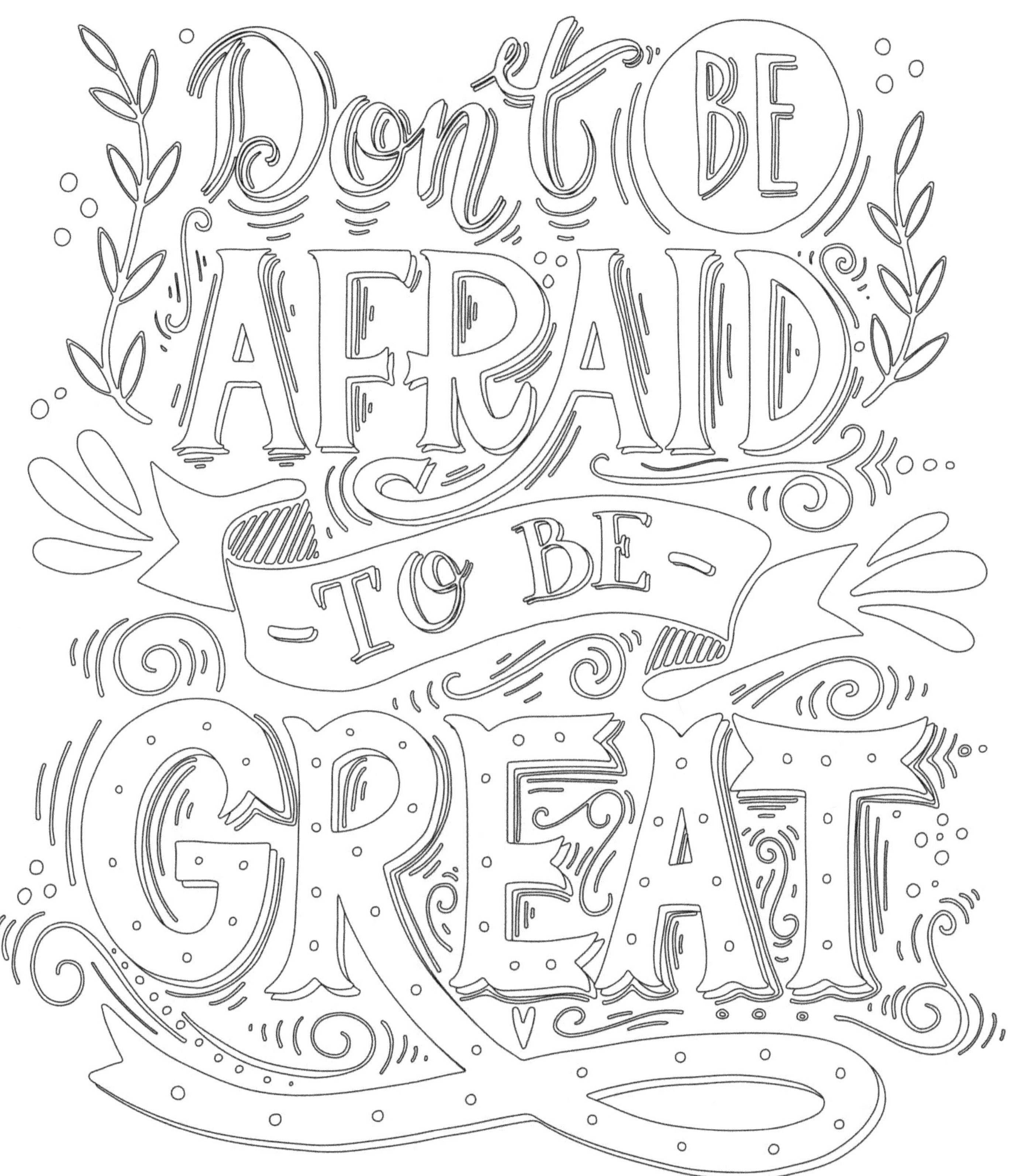
Don't BE
AFRAID
- TO BE -
GREAT

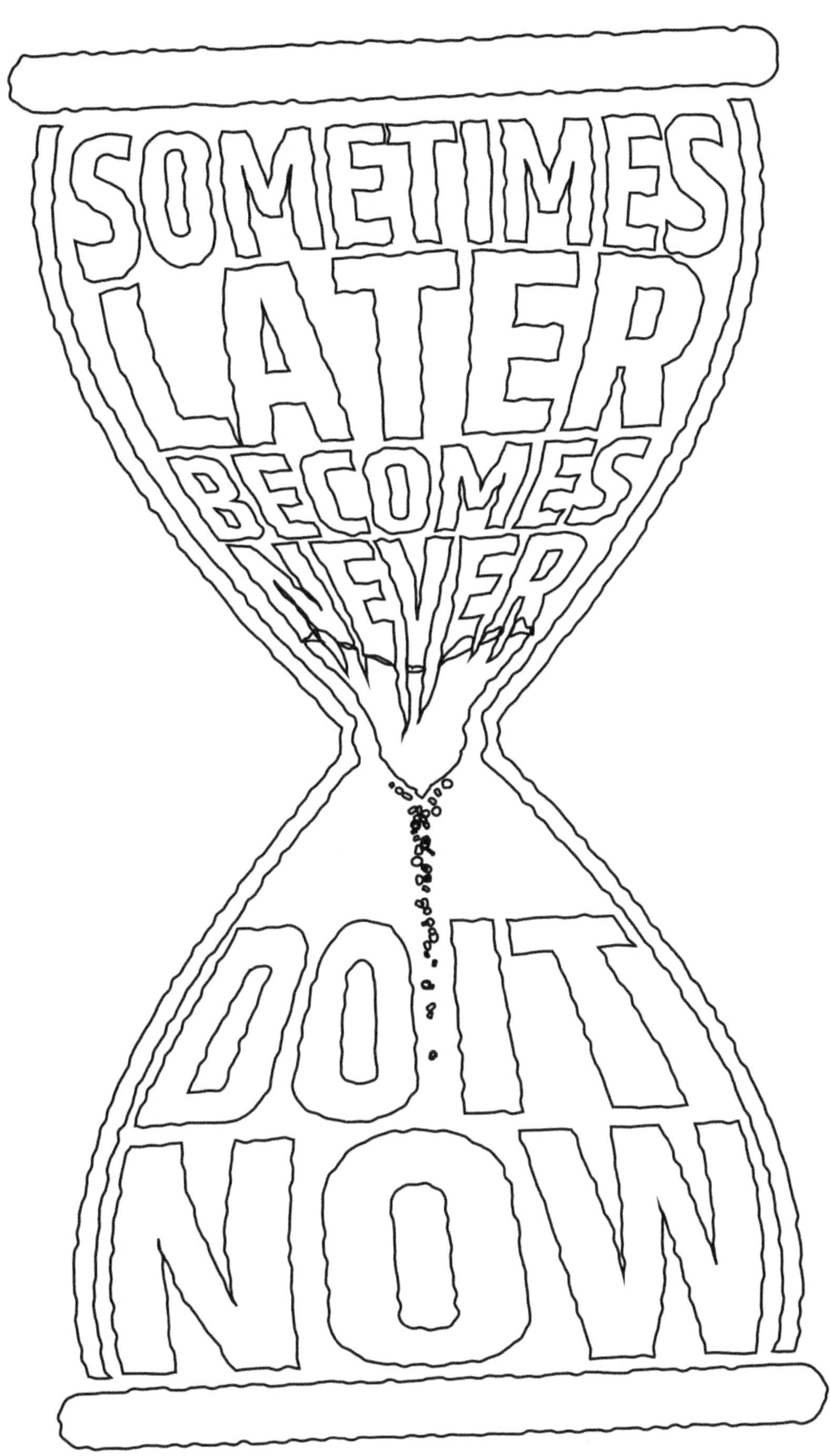

SOMETIMES
LATER
BECOMES
NEVER
DO IT
NOW

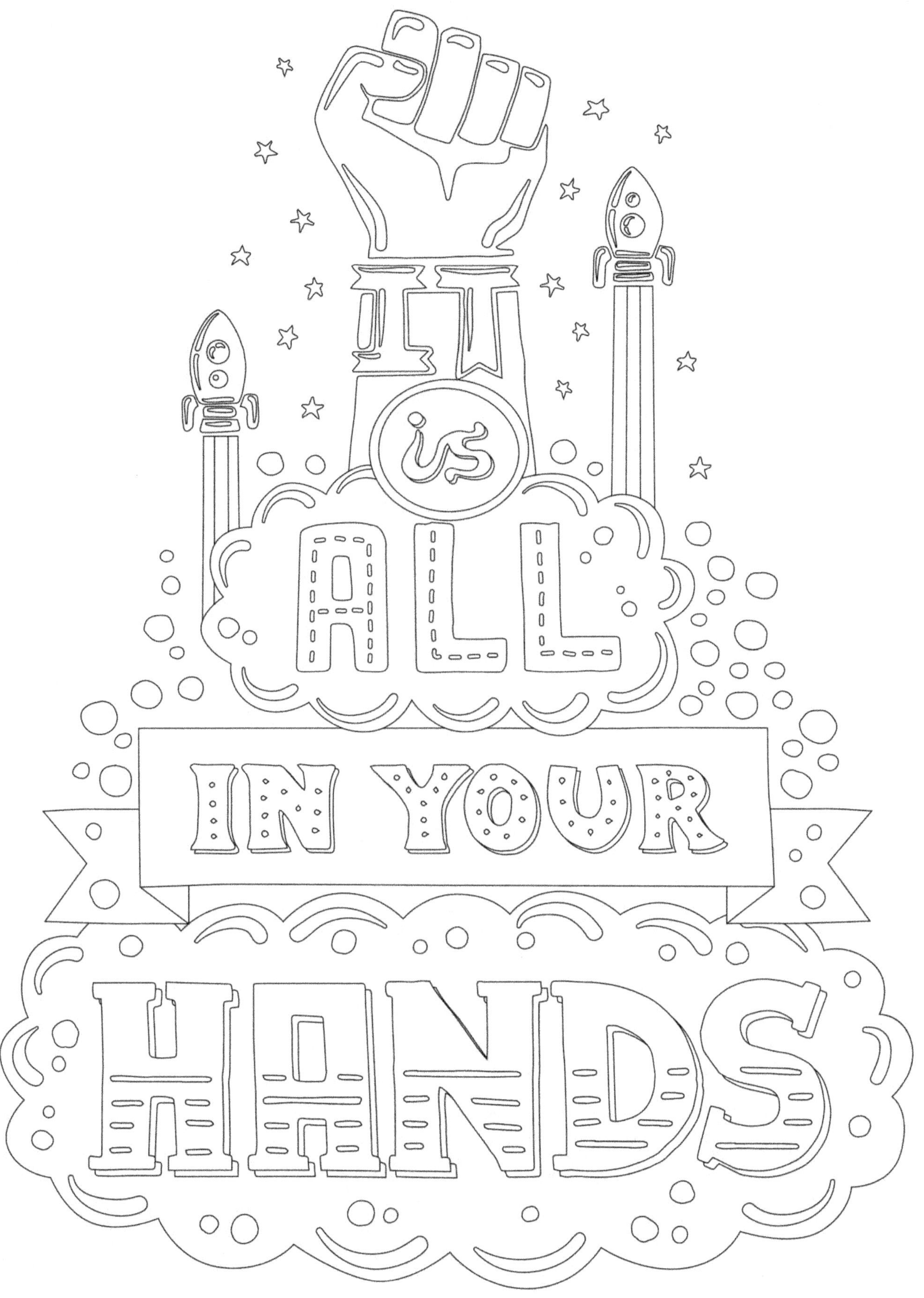
IT
IS
ALL
IN YOUR
HANDS

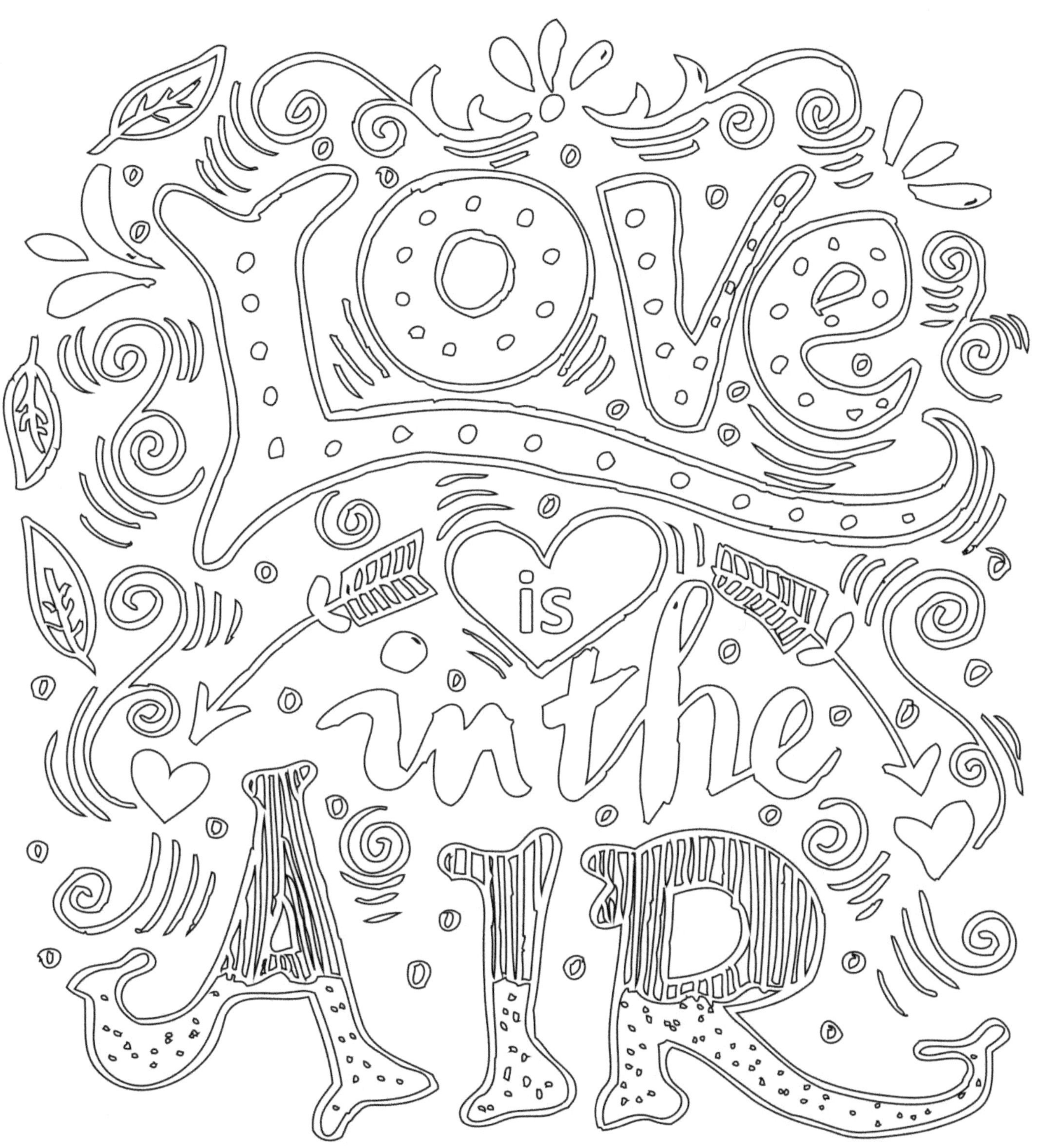

LOVE
is
in the
AIR

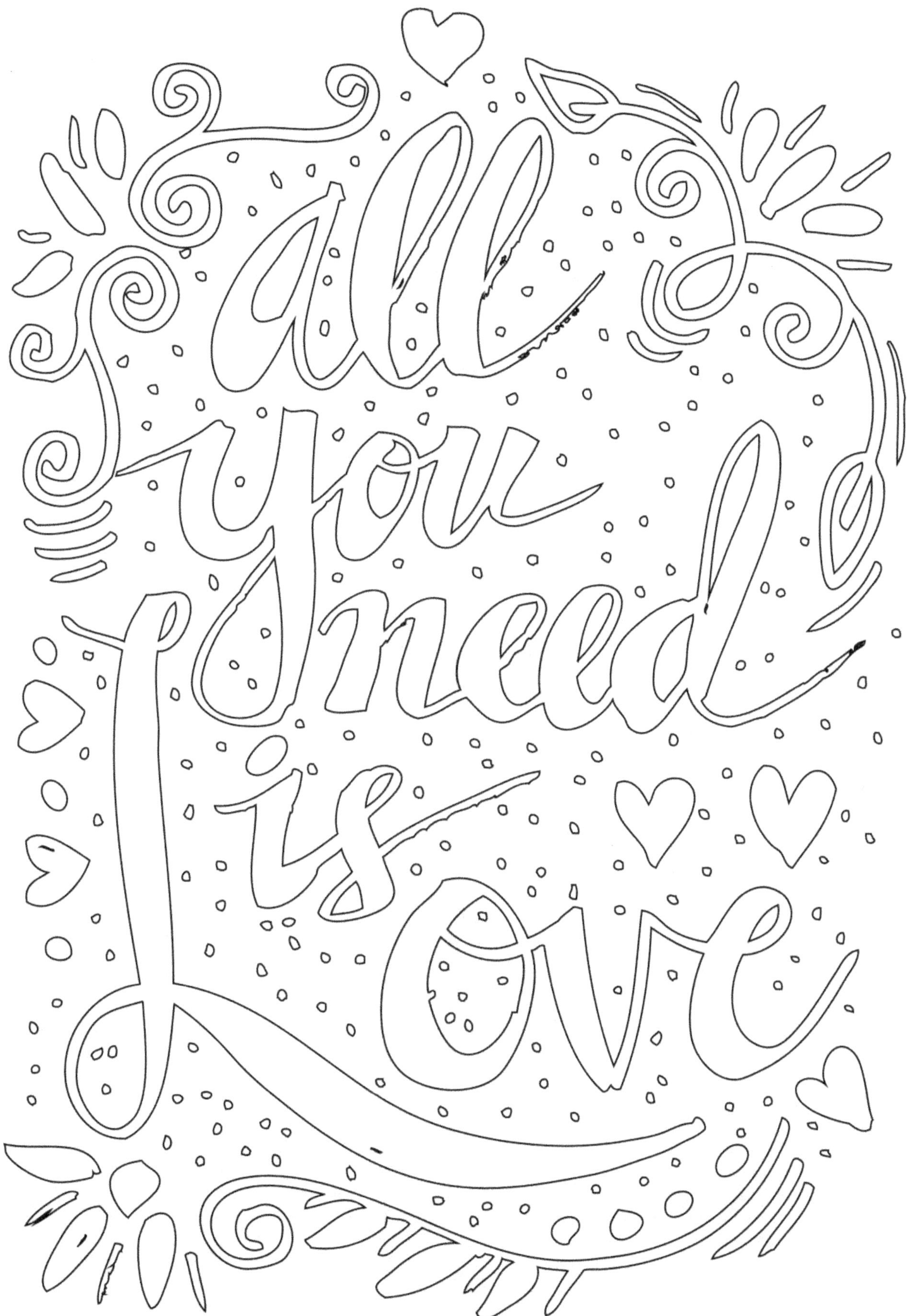
all
you
need
is
Love

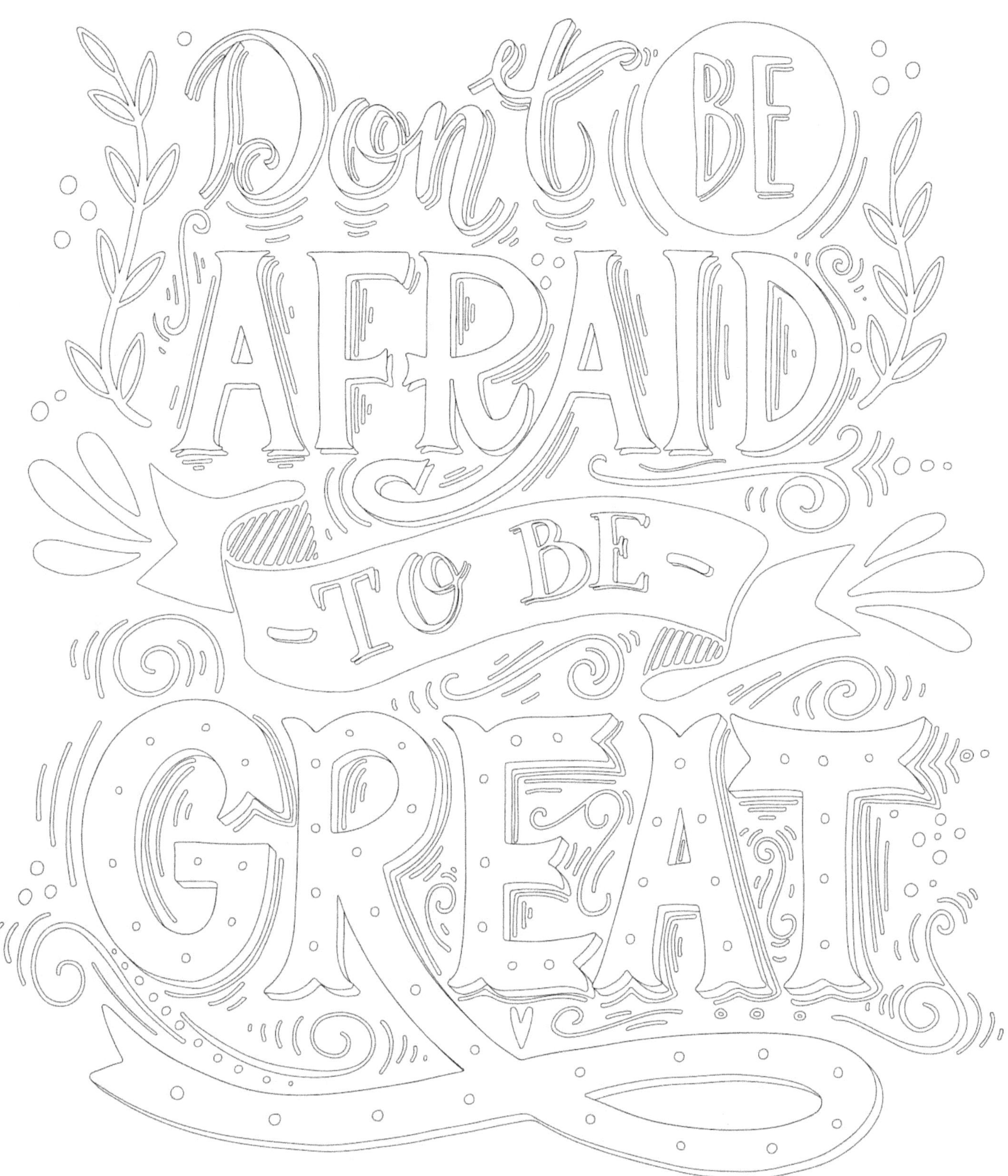
Don't BE AFRAID
- TO BE -
GREAT

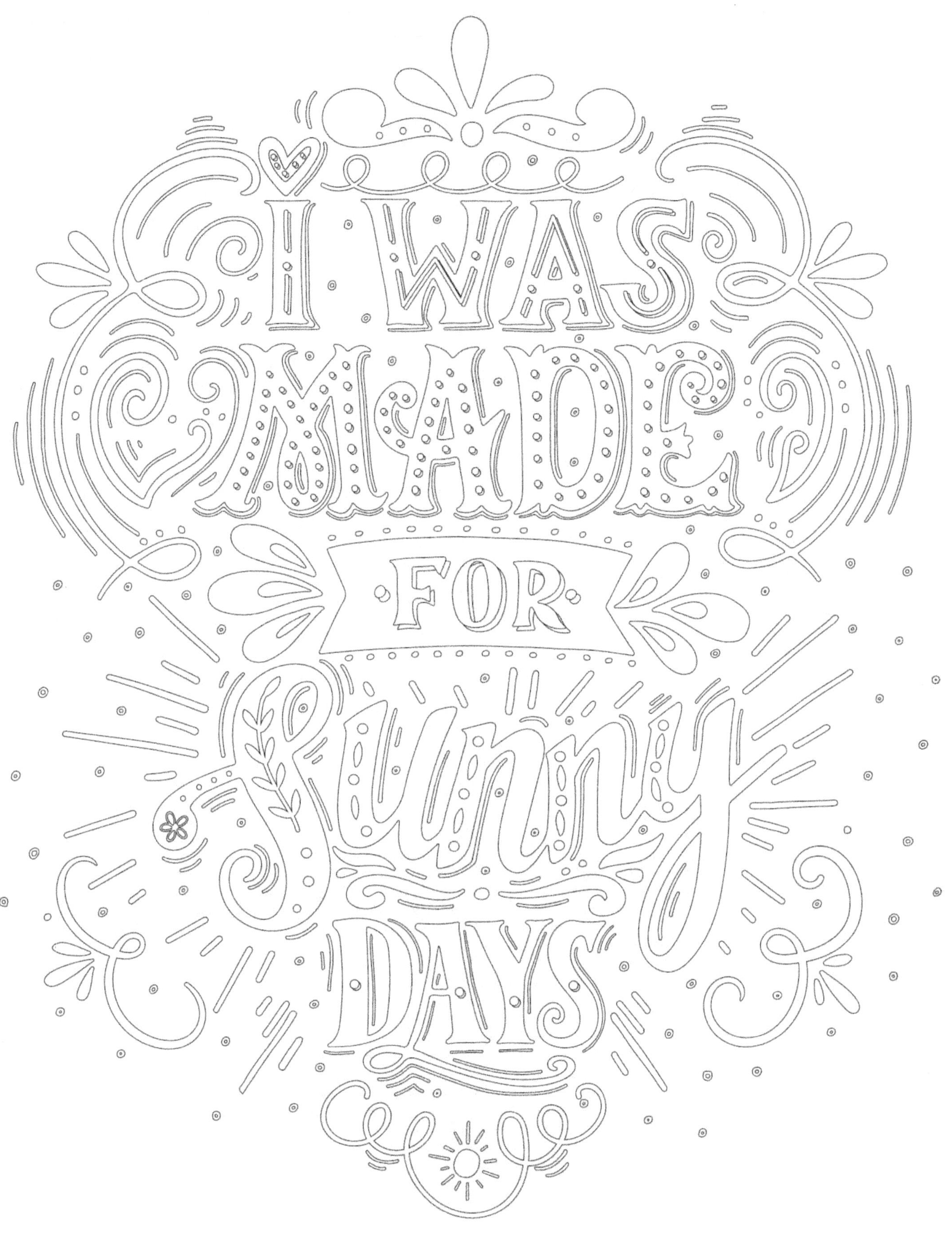
I WAS MADE FOR SUNNY DAYS

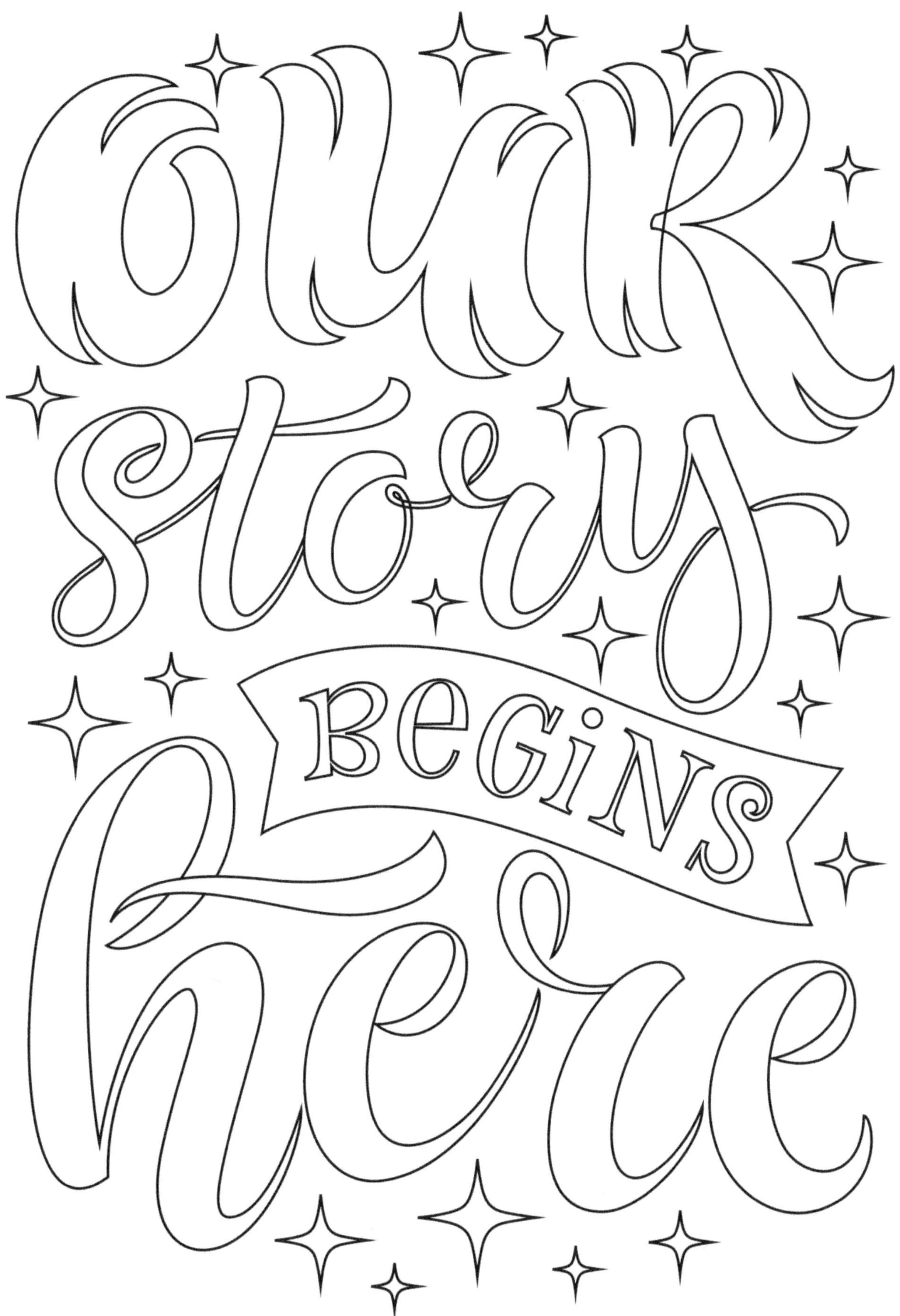

OUR
story
BEGINS
here

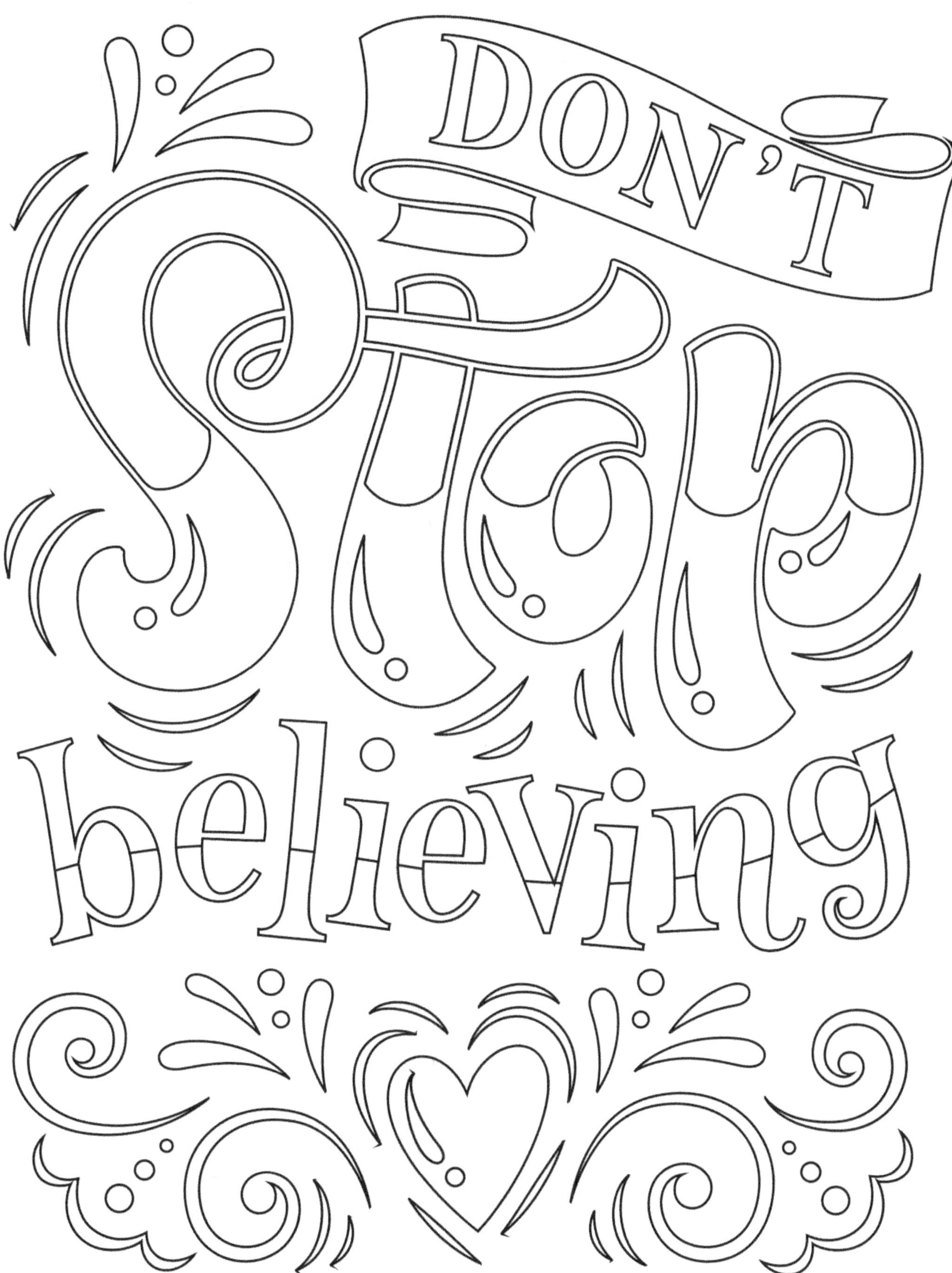

Don't
Stop
believing

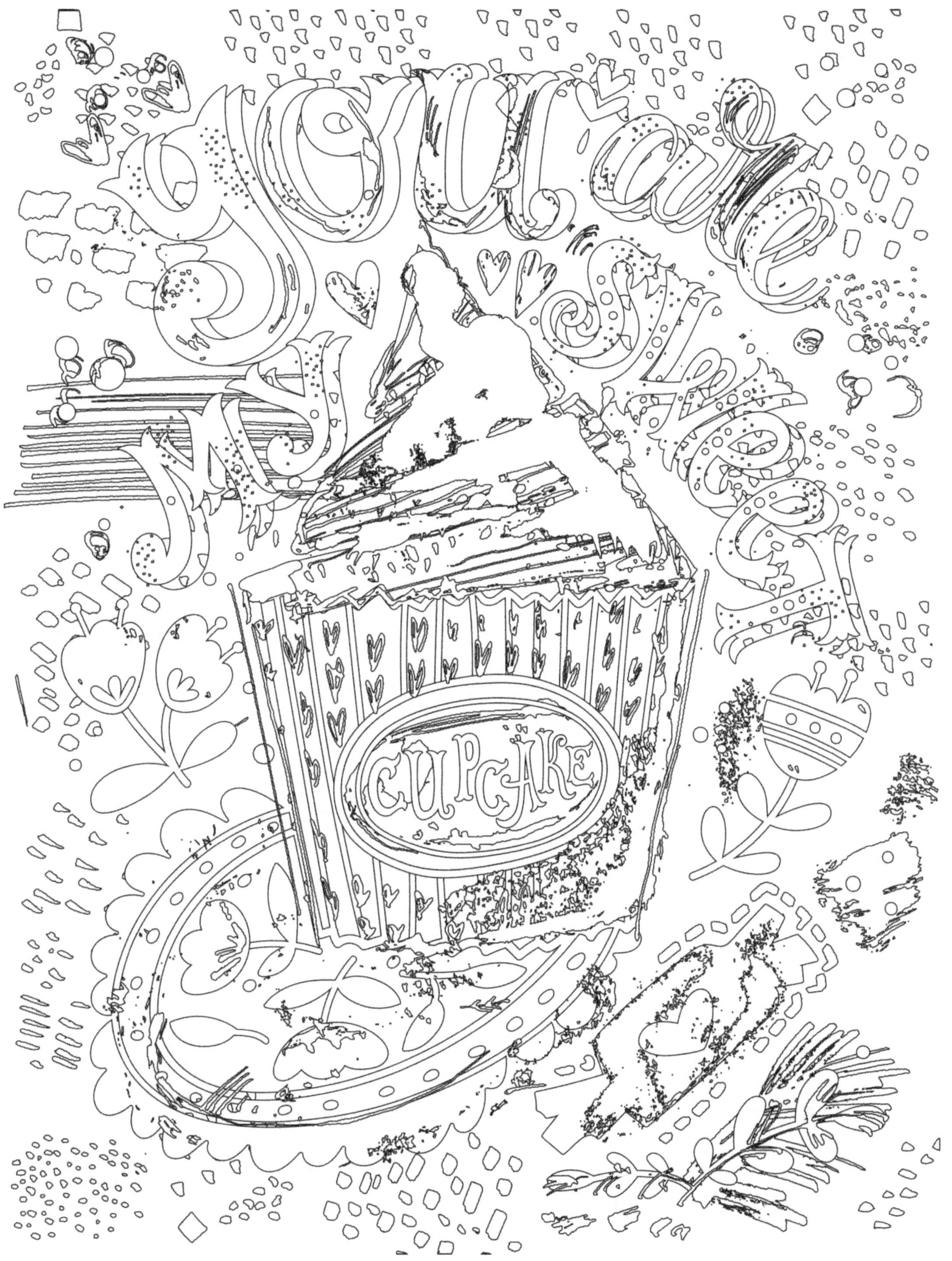

You are as sweet
CUPCAKE

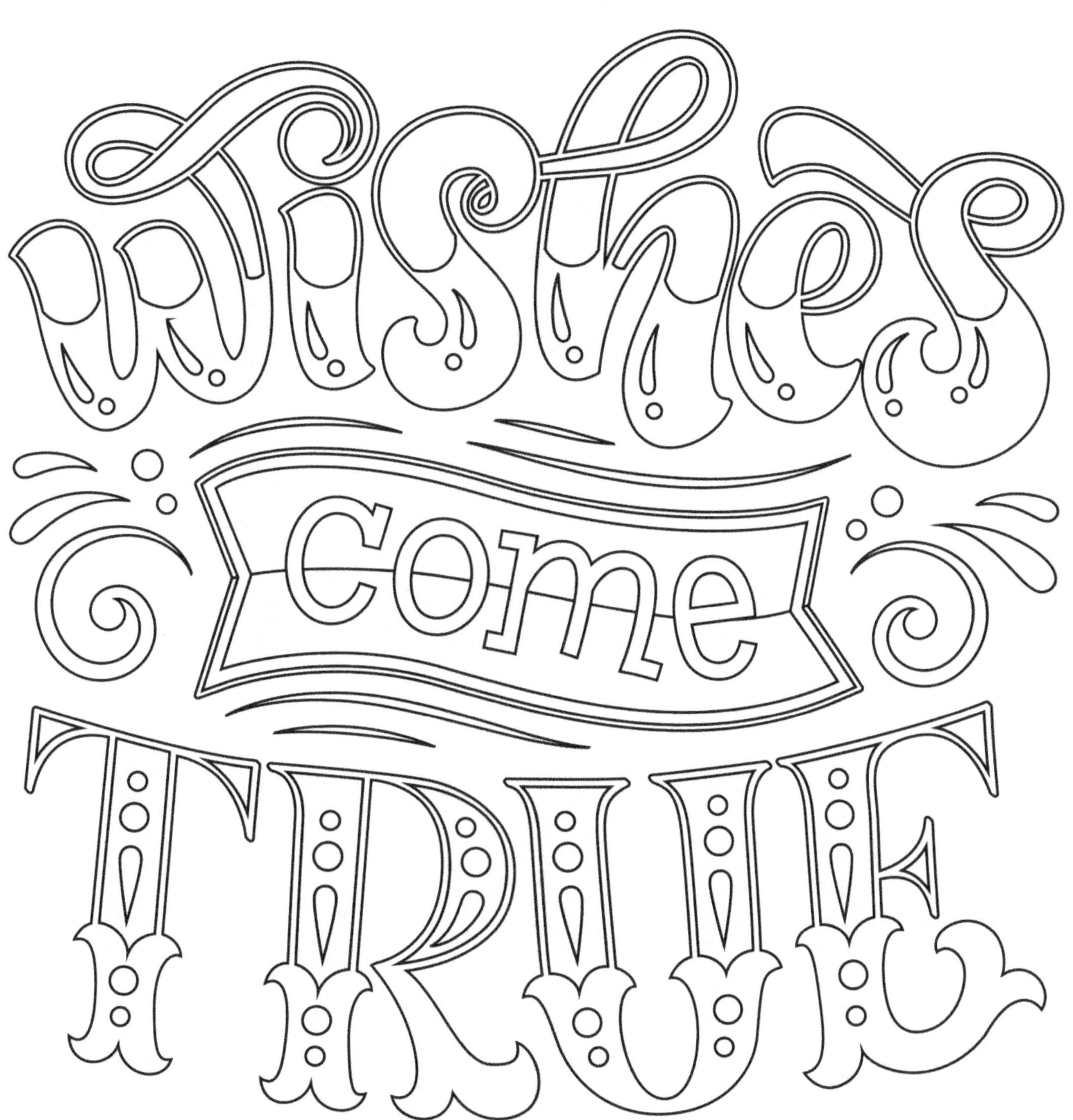

Wishes
come
TRUE

Sleep less & Dream more

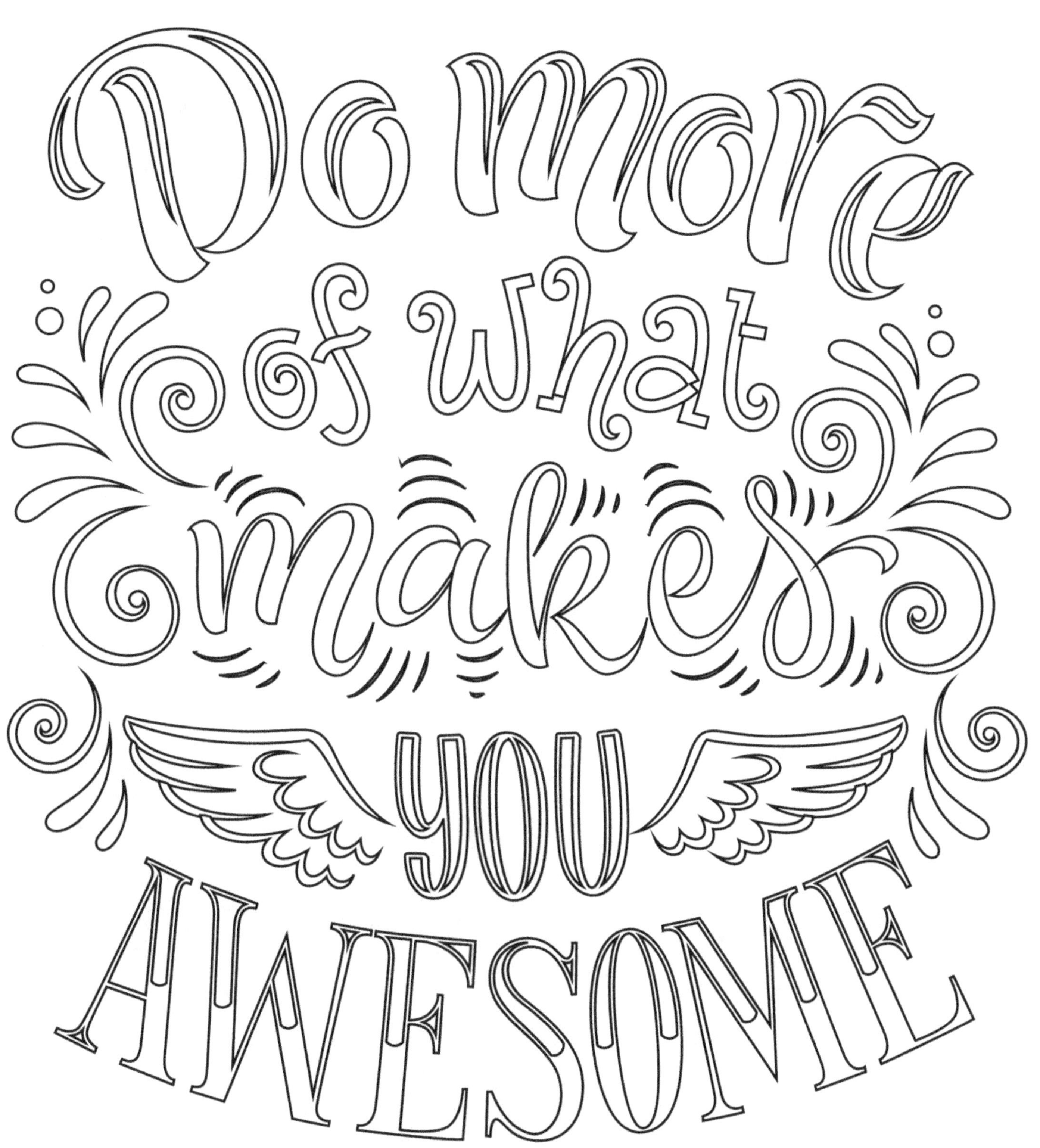

Do more
of what
makes
you
AWESOME

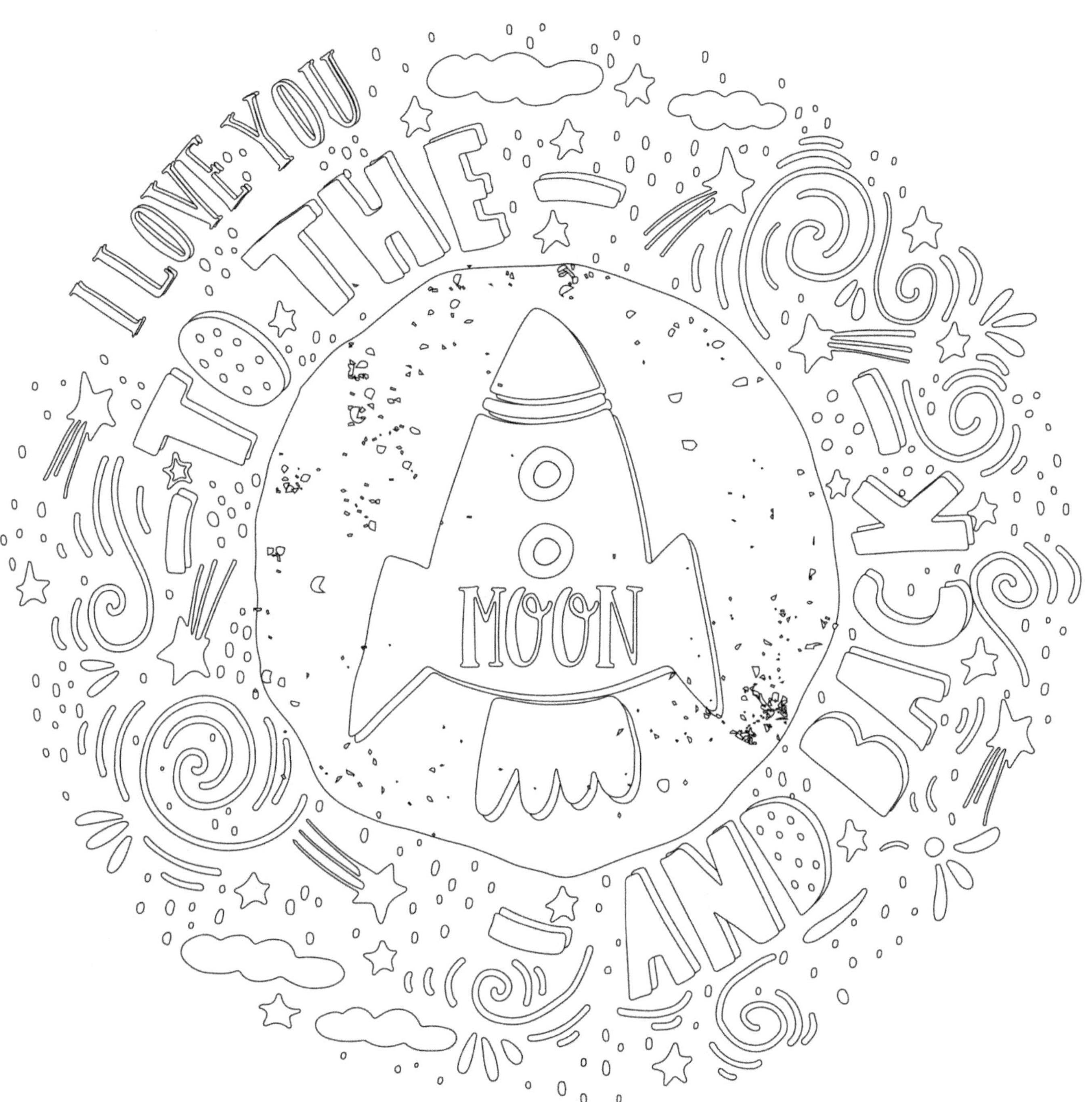

I LOVE YOU
TO THE
MOON
AND BACK

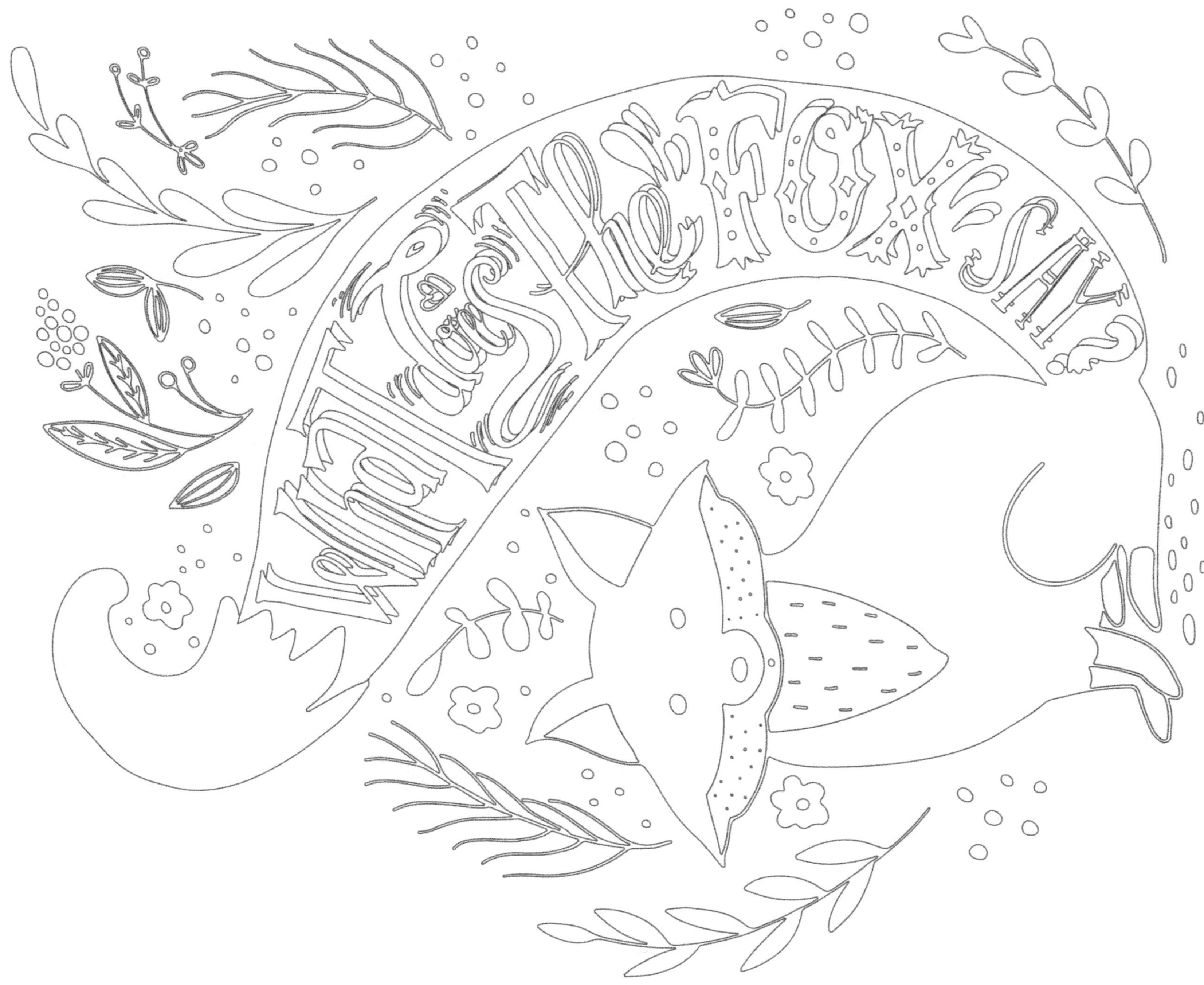
What Does The Fox Say

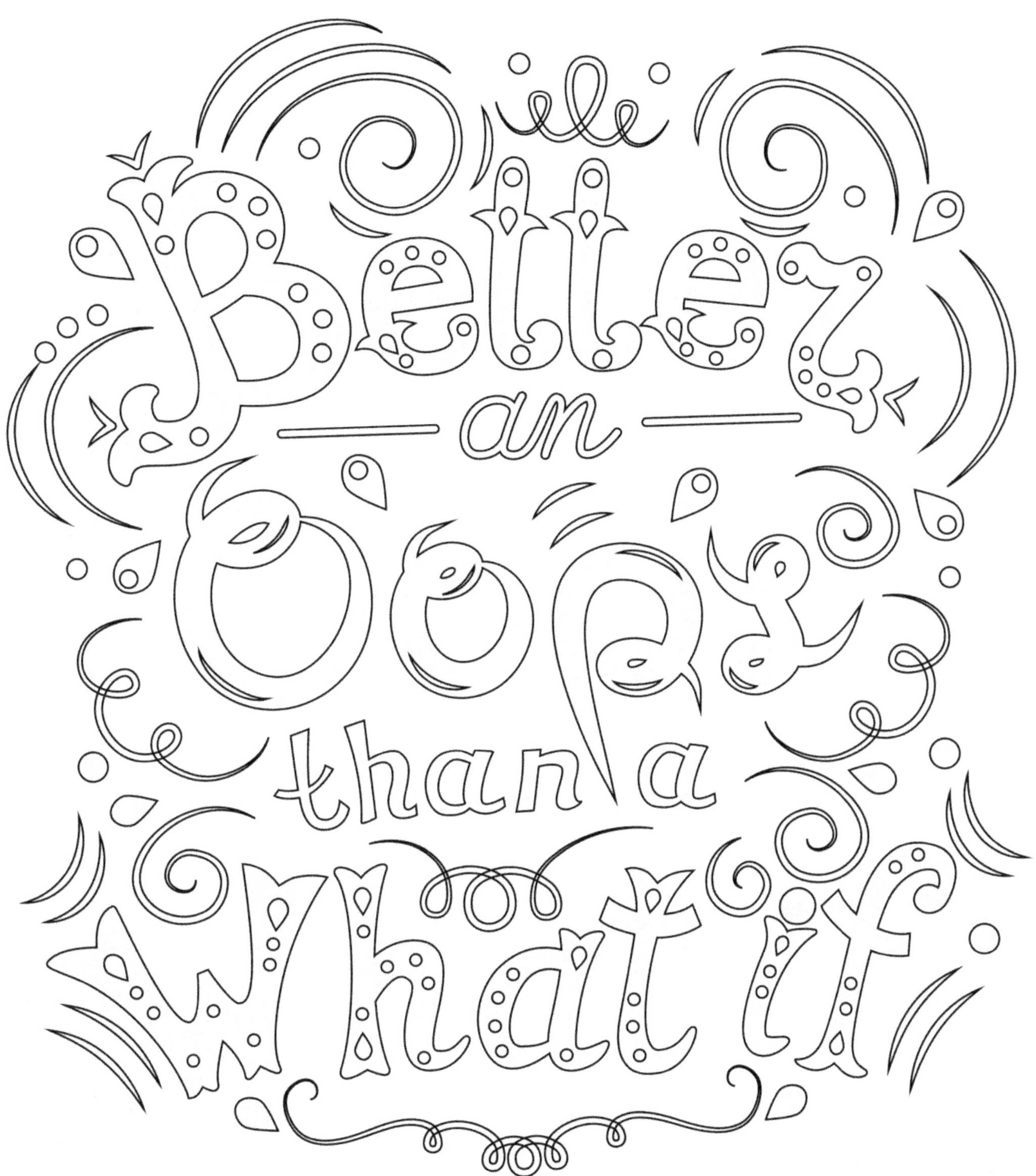

Better
an
oops
than a
what if

www.ingramcontent.com/pod-product-compliance
Lightning Source LLC
Chambersburg PA
CBHW080815280726
48660CB00018B/3464